Optimize Your Life Series— Book 2

The Sleep Habit

Simple, Natural, and Healthy Steps to Sleep Like a Baby in Just 3 Days

ISBN: 978-1-7369687-2-7

Acknowledgements

Thank you for supporting me as I wrote book 2! I greatly appreciate my family and friends for all of their help. And thank you again to Sara Pack, fastest-editor-in-the-west! She can be reached at SaraPackEditing.com.

Contents

Basics of Sleep

Your body has a twenty-four-hour clock called a circadian rhythm. Your body's clock is regulated by exposure to light, exercise, nutrients, and hormones. When it is working well, you experience wakefulness during daylight and sleepiness during nighttime. Your body naturally produces melatonin, and its levels peak about two hours before bedtime. Your body's wake-up juice is the hormone cortisol.

Melatonin

As I mentioned above, your body produces melatonin naturally. I should say most bodies produce the optimum levels of melatonin naturally. There are ways to boost your melatonin through food, supplements, exposure to sunlight, and exercise.

There are several ways to screw up your body's ability to produce melatonin, such as exposure to the blue light emitted from screens. Inconsistent sleep and wake times and eating or drinking too late at night are also fabulous ways to mess up your melatonin levels.

Finally, the granddaddy of barriers to melatonin production is stress! Basically, stress produces cortisol, which is your body's wake-up juice. Just like most of us wouldn't drink a cup of coffee right before bed, we shouldn't play an adrenaline-inducing game, for example, right before bed, as this floods us with cortisol.

Cortisol

I think of cortisol as it relates to stress. Too much stress equals too much cortisol, which means I need to meditate or exercise or journal to get myself back to normal. However, cortisol is a naturally occurring hormone that helps regulate the wake-up period of our circadian rhythm. This is why cortisol levels are naturally higher in the morning.

Cortisol is used in a variety of other functions, including:

- blood sugar regulation,
- inflammation reduction,
- metabolism regulation, and
- memory formulation.

Hmmm, is it beginning to make sense how our sleep difficulties can have so much of an adverse effect on our health, weight, diabetes, etc.? Cortisol also fuels our fight-or-flight response in an emergency. That is *not* something we want to trigger when we are trying to get to sleep.

To reduce levels of cortisol, start a gratitude journal before bed. Writing about stressful experiences will increase cortisol, but writing about positive experiences or even planning for the next day will lower your levels. Relaxing bedtime activities also include listening to music or caring for a pet. Knowing the circumstances that increase cortisol and the actions you can take to lower cortisol is just one brick in the sleep habit foundation we will build together.

Introduction

Up until I began my chosen career path, I slept great. In college, I was playing volleyball, getting good grades, working, and going to school at night, and I was able to sleep pretty darn well. And I LOVE to sleep. Give me my comfy bed and even comfier body pillow (seriously, why do they not become a thing until pregnancy?), and I will sleep in like a teenager!

However, I have developed quite the problem falling asleep. What should I do? Medication? "Oh, by the way, this is highly addictive." No thank you.

Well, maybe. It really depends on how many nights it's been since I felt like I slept.

Did you know that not sleeping is actually a great way to drive yourself insane? No really, serious torture techniques involve no sleep. Prisoners can't tell what's reality. It's pretty horrible stuff. Don't google that.

Okay, so now that you're back from that rabbit hole (I warned you!), what can you do to develop good sleep habits? Well, you can go talk to your medical doctor, or you can go talk to a therapist.

I actually recommend both of those steps. I also want to give you a step-by-step guide to follow *in addition to* the professional help that I recommended above. When you are not sleeping well, complicated stuff does not make sense. Easy things seem as complicated as preparing to climb Mt. Everest, so why try? Here are some simple, easy-to-take steps that cost very little money and can totally revamp your sleep habits in just three days. Seriously.

However, this isn't a choose-your-own-adventure guide. You will need to actually act on every step. If there are choices, I will let you know. Otherwise, EVERY step must happen.

Mindset

Okay, I really hope you have read *The Shower Habit* because this will make so much more sense if you have. However, if you haven't, I will break it down for you here:

- Mindset matters.
- Read about Carol Dweck.
- Your belief is your truth.

Carol Dweck coined the term "growth mindset" to describe people who believe that with hard work and perseverance, you can learn and grow.

This will work if you follow the steps, even talking to your doctor and therapist, and you *believe* it will work. If you are a serious skeptic, no worries. Your homework is to take the quiz. Make ALL the changes suggested. Read this book once and put it away for a week. Then re-read the book and follow every step. Your mind has to see the possibilities before you begin. This technique of giving yourself time to process the information will help with most habits that you want to start. You just need time to convince your brain that this can work. Get your Negative Nelly inner voice on board and go for it! Serious skeptics may need more than three days for this new sleep habit to work, but it will still work!

To make this easier to implement, I have divided this book into three parts. Parts I and III are super easy to implement. Like most things in life, though, the easy changes are not where the most growth happens. Part II is the magic of your new and improved sleep habit. This is not going to be easy, but it is simple and will make a huge difference in your quality and quantity of sleep.

Importance of Sleep

Sleep is really important for health and being on top of your game. Attention, problem solving, and reflexes are all tied to getting enough sleep. Also, a lack of sleep is tied to numerous health conditions like obesity, type 2 diabetes, high blood pressure, heart disease, stroke, poor mental health, and even early death. Yikes! Early death is not something we need, so get good sleep by implementing effective routines.

The Premise & Quiz

As so many people have sleep issues, I decided to do some research, purely for the benefit of the masses. Really, it had nothing to do with the fact that I couldn't sleep. Nothing.

Is sleeping a skill? Can we all "get good" at sleep? Why do some people struggle so much?

If you are anything like me—and I say that with a wry grin—you like to know how things work. I really like to know the theory behind everything. However, I am not the take-the-engine-apart-to-learn-about-it type of gal. I am the type who reads the research, buys the books, watches the videos, and downloads the audiobooks. Then I want to find someone who knows a lot about the topic so I can ask a million questions.

Yep, I'm annoying like that. However, that quality is going to allow you to find the relevant information about sleep right here in this short book. Because after I synthesize the heaps of information, I can summarize it down to the bare bones.

Did you read *The Shower Habit*? That is a ton of information on starting your day off successfully, all pared-down to under eighty pages. You can even listen to the audio if you don't like to read. It's packed with super helpful stuff that I want you to try.

It's the same with this book. I truly believe that happy people make our entire world better. Sleeping better and starting your day off right will lead you to be a happier person, and that has a domino effect that helps us all.

Another deep reason that I began my search for all things sleep-related has to do with being a breast cancer survivor. There is a really strong correlation between being a cancer survivor and having sleep issues. That is not cool. After beating cancer, survivors should be able to get a good night's sleep.

Okay, back to the research. How many sleep disorders have been identified?

A. 10
B. 25
C. Over 50
D. Over 100

Yes, it's D for the win! Amazingly, over one hundred different sleep disorders have been documented. Basically, they are categorized into one or more of the following:

- trouble falling or remaining asleep
- difficulty staying awake during the day
- imbalances in the circadian rhythm that interfere with a healthy sleep schedule
- unusual behaviors that disrupt sleep

With over a hundred sleep disorders out there, people have done some outrageous things while sleeping—driving a car, eating, gardening naked, and more. My favorite is the story of a guy who woke up in the morning and opened a cupboard in his kitchen to find that he had completely filled each and every cup, bowl, and dish with water. Each dish was full to the very top! While some of the stories are pretty comical, can you imagine waking up with dirty feet and having no idea where you had been?

Unfortunately, this book is not designed to cure those with diagnosed sleep disorders. This book is designed to provide tips, based on research, that in some combination will work to improve your ability to fall asleep, stay asleep, and feel rested when you wake up.

As more and more people complain about having trouble sleeping, if you listen, they usually suspect a specific reason for their sleep difficulties. You will hear that their sleep troubles are due to:

- work stress,
- worry about kids/family,
- eating habits (usually spicy food or caffeine),
- uncomfortable bed,
- hormones,
- side effects of medication, or
- if they are lucky, simply a really good book!

In many cases, I suspect the variables are so many that pinpointing one cause would be impossible. The great news is, even if all the underlying issues are not totally resolved, most of the time, you can experience relief in sleep difficulties.

I am deeply sorry about the sleep issues you are experiencing. It is so complicated. And it involves an unidentified epidemic happening in our world today. Over 40 percent of the population is getting fewer than seven hours of sleep per night. A surprising 60–80 percent of high school students report fewer than eight hours of sleep per night.

Researchers asked the question: Is our sleep getting worse? The basic answer was yes! In every category measured, more people are now being diagnosed with sleep disorders.

Hmmm, I wonder what fabulous invention is now in everyone's hands that wasn't readily available just twenty years ago....

Psychology of Behavior Change

Let's take a little bird walk here. In our world currently, most everybody knows and acknowledges that reading to your kids is beneficial. Does everybody know and acknowledge that having a tech-free family dinner is beneficial? How about the no-tech-before-bed rule?

I know, I know, kale is good for you too, but I do not want to eat it with every meal. Just because we know something doesn't mean that our actions follow our knowledge.

That's where the amazing benefits of habits come in. A habit does not require you to think or make a decision. A habit is just something you do. It becomes a part of who you are. I am a reader. I love to read. Reading is a habit, a hobby, and an activity that I enjoy. Reading is also a habit that has some pretty good benefits and not too many downsides. So, I am keeping that habit.

Lead vs. Lag

Have you heard about the difference in lead versus lag measures when it comes to tracking progress toward your goals? If not, I highly suggest you read a book titled, *The Four Disciplines of Execution: Achieving Your Wildly Important Goals* by Sean Covey. In this book, the author explains that one of the reasons we set goals and fail so often is that we track the wrong data.

In an effort to achieve a healthier weight, we track how much we weigh. The number of pounds we weigh is a lag measure, meaning that it is the result of other factors. If we track the calories we eat or the minutes we exercise, those measures lead to the lag measure of how much we weigh. So, if we want to impact the lag measure, our weight, we should really be tracking the calories we eat or even the number of nights we lay out our exercise clothes to prepare to exercise the next morning, which are lead measures. Even better, we should be tracking the groceries we buy and the meals we plan and prep. That's a super lead measure.

To take this into the realm of quality sleep, the number of hours of sleep we get each night is the lag measure. We need to figure out the best lead measures that will result in better sleep. It will depend on our individual bodies, but we will be able to figure it out. It could be tracking steps, bedtime routines, or the amount of time between the last time we picked up our phone and bedtime.

What will work for you will be different than what works for me. But the good news is, we know all the possible ingredients. We just need to write the perfect recipe for you.

Bed Quiz

Let's start with your setup. If your environment isn't comfortable, how can you be? If you can't check off every item below, stop reading now. Making a few simple changes might give you results right away!

- ☐ My sheets have been washed in the last two weeks.
- ☐ My bed has only bedding on it.
- ☐ There are no laundry baskets or piles of clothes in my bedroom.
- ☐ I have a nightstand with a lamp.
- ☐ I have a journal, pen, lip balm, and nail file on or in my nightstand.
- ☐ I like my pillow and pillowcase.

Now that you have checked every item above, you may continue to Part I of your new sleep habit.

Part I
The Prep

The first step in the sleep habit that will help us feel energetic and rested has everything to do with how we fuel our bodies. What foods are we putting in? Do these foods lead to the outcomes we want?

Chapter 1—Food List

Melatonin: a hormone made by the pineal gland (tiny organ near the center of the brain). Melatonin helps control the body's sleep cycle and is an antioxidant. It is also made in the laboratory and sold as a supplement.
—from the National Cancer Institute

Have you heard the saying, "You are what you eat"? Well, our new saying is #eat4sleep. Maybe I need to work on that. Or maybe it works. I just looked it up on Twitter and found that two people have used that hashtag. Sweet!

Okay, back to the saying that you are what you eat. There are four main vitamins and minerals found in food that aid in promoting sleep—tryptophan, magnesium, calcium, and B6. Let's be really clear. I am not a doctor, nor do I play one on TV. You should talk to your doctor about adding to or changing your diet. The entire point of this book is to help you feel better. Your doctor needs to be part of that wellness team. You need to be an educated part of that team, and this book is one component to help you get educated about yourself and your sleep.

Tryptophan and B6

Tryptophan is an amino acid found in many foods that can help your body make the hormone melatonin. Tryptophan is used by the body to make serotonin, and it is then turned into melatonin.

However, if you are low in B6, your body has a harder time turning tryptophan into melatonin. So, in order for your body to do this efficiently, you need B6. Read through the following lists and then go stock up on a few of these items.

> Foods containing Tryptophan:
> - Dairy—milk, cheese, yogurt
> - Fruits—apples, peaches, bananas, avocados
> - Seeds—pumpkin, sesame, sunflower, flax,
> - Nuts—walnuts, almonds, peanuts, cashews
> - Vegetables—broccoli, spinach, asparagus, onion
> - Seafood and poultry—tuna, shrimp, salmon, sardines, cod, turkey, chicken

> Foods containing B6 (remember, your body needs B6 to help convert tryptophan):
> - Seeds—sunflower, flax
> - Nuts—pistachio
> - Seafood and meat—tuna, salmon, halibut, chicken, pork, beef
> - Fruit—banana, avocado, dried prunes
> - Vegetables—spinach

Magnesium

Magnesium is a mineral that naturally relaxes the body and helps deactivate adrenaline. I need that on hand when my kids jump out to scare me before bed! Or maybe I need to feed it to my kids and husband because I hide in their dark bedrooms and jump out to scare them too. Whatever. It's because I love them.

- ➤ Foods containing Magnesium:
  - Dairy—yogurt
  - Seeds—sunflower, flax
  - Nuts—cashews, brazil nuts, pecans
  - Fruits—bananas, avocados
  - Vegetables—baby spinach, kale, dark leafy greens
  - Seafood—salmon, halibut, tuna, mackerel

Relaxing muscles helps not only with sleep but also with constipation. And that helps our gut bacteria, which is very pertinent to our overall health.

Calcium

Calcium also helps your body make melatonin. Remember, making melatonin is good, as this hormone helps you get to sleep and stay asleep.

- ➤ Foods containing Calcium:
  - Dairy—milk, cheese, yogurt
  - Vegetables—green snap peas, okra, broccoli
  - Seafood—sardines

Melatonin

Now that we have covered all the foods that can help your body with sleep, primarily by being turned into melatonin, we will look at the foods that are excellent sources of naturally occurring melatonin.

- ➢ Foods containing melatonin:
  - Seeds—sunflower, mustard, flax
  - Nuts—walnuts, peanuts
  - Fruits—tart cherries, pomegranate, grapes, tomatoes
  - Vegetables—corn, asparagus, olives, broccoli, cucumber

Based on that entire list of foods that will help me sleep, I am thinking a nice yogurt with cherries, walnuts, and sunflower seeds might be the perfect evening food. The only problem is most yogurt has way too much sugar. Spiking our blood sugar is not helpful for so many reasons. One, a spike in sugar increases energy. Two, the crash from the sugar high causes hunger. So maybe a trail mix of walnuts, peanuts, sunflower seeds, cherries, and dried prunes would be a better idea.

Instead of trying to add sleep-friendly foods to your diet one at a time, why not eat sleep-friendly dinners? Plan an entire week of meals that will help you sleep, and eat at least two or three hours before bedtime. Give your food a chance to get at least part of the way through your digestive tract before you lie down. Keep reading for a few slumber-inducing dinner ideas.

➤ Sleepy Food Meals:
- Salmon, asparagus
- Almond-crusted halibut with tomato, onion, cucumber salad
- Cheddar broccoli soup
- Tuna avocado melt
- Pomegranate avocado toast
- Caramelized onion and cherry tartine

If this idea of weekly sleepy food dinners sounds intriguing, head on over to my website at stephanieewingauthor.com and sign up to download the four-week sleep food dinner recipe booklet. This is free, so go grab it!

Tip

Whether you want to focus on foods that help your body create melatonin, foods that naturally contain melatonin, or supplements that give your body melatonin, any of these choices will work. But you need to consistently get melatonin into your body! If you have been experiencing sleep challenges, you need to keep melatonin as an integral part of your newly created sleep habit.

Chapter 2—Clutter Serene

Serene: Marked by or suggestive of utter calm and unruffled repose or quietude.
—from Merriam-Webster

You can buy entire books on decluttering your house—I have read many of them! For sleeping, let's just focus on the bedroom for now. If you want to tackle your entire house, that's great! But let's not start that right before bed, mmkay?

Also, there are books that have you start by emptying the entire space and only putting back what is going to stay. That is a great idea if you have a totally empty spare room or if your garage is spick and span and empty. Yep, that idea is great for a very, very small number of us.

The idea of making one space better by making another space worse doesn't make a whole lotta sense for me. Yes, if you were able to get an entire space empty and put back only the things that you desire to keep, all in one day by yourself with no interruptions, that might work. I do not happen to know people like that. My friends all have jobs, pets, kids, friends and family, hobbies, stamina issues, attention challenges, or other commitments that usually take precedence over that kind of all-day session.

Instead, I advocate for a process that does not make another mess as it happens. Focus on one tiny area, such as the top of your nightstand. Having a functional, clean, clutter-free nightstand, along with a garbage can, next to your bed is essential for this new sleep habit we are co-creating. These along with a dirty-clothes hamper are necessary items in your bedroom and will allow you to keep it clutter free and serene.

Clutter Serene

Messy sleep is rough. Usually, our sleep challenges have a complicated origin, so it takes a precise recipe of actions to see relief. Unfortunately, there aren't any one-step answers, and I'm all out of magic pixie dust.

One ingredient for happy sleep is having a clutter-free sleeping space. I can tell you from my own experience that surroundings are a huge part of my successful sleep habit.

Go to the space where you sleep and look at the space right around your bed. Do you have a nightstand? What's on it? Do you have a dresser or chair or clothes rack (aka treadmill) in your bedroom? These are all fine as long as you can see their tops. If the space looks or feels cluttered, let's work on that one step at a time.

Start with your nightstand. Take everything off and clean the top of it. Then very carefully decide what will go back. I do not recommend a lot of pictures or knick-knacks. Stick with a lamp, journal, and something to write with. If you must keep one other item on your nightstand, make it something that evokes a peaceful, serene feeling.

Next up, look down at the floor in your sleeping area. Pick up any items on the floor and sweep, vacuum, and/or mop the floor. The action of cleaning the nightstand and the floor is enough for right now. In the coming weeks, tackle any other organizing, minimalizing, or beautification projects in this space.

My best resource for organizing is *Decluttering at the Speed of Life* by Dana K. White. This practical read has all the elements that I advocate for a happier home in terms of tidiness. The process is practical and can be accomplished one tiny space at a time without creating other messes to clean up in the future.

Tip

Before we leave the area, look at the light in the room. Do your curtains or window coverings block out the light? If you are not able to sleep because the sun is out, please work on getting your bedroom very dark for your sleep time. Light really can affect your ability to fall asleep and stay asleep.

You may be very skeptical of these recommendations, but remember, the success of your sleep habit will depend on multiple variables. This might not seem like a huge change, but the cumulative effects can lead to a world of difference in your life!

Chapter 3—Sleeping Surface

Memory Foam: a polyurethane material that is sensitive to pressure and temperature, used especially in mattresses, where it molds to the shape of an individual's body.
—from Oxford Languages

Have you ever watched *The Blindside*? In the movie, a previously homeless teenage football player is taken to his new room, and he says, "I've never had one before." His new mom says, "What, a bedroom to yourself?" He answers, "No, a bed."

Sleeping on couches or the floor is not ideal. I am sure we have all experienced a comfortable couch or recliner, but night after night? This is not a long-term solution to sleep challenges. To have our minds fully on board with this new sleep habit, we need to be able to assign a space to this habit. If you must sleep in a one-room type situation, create a sense of boundaries between spaces. This could be hanging curtains or placing a room divider or plant stand. Just have something that delineates the space for sleeping. Then only use that space for sleeping (or sex). No watching TV or playing on your phone in your bed.

Mattress

Finding the perfect mattress for you to sleep on can be difficult. However, I think many of us can sleep on a variety of mattresses if the rest of our sleep habit is solid. My hypothesis is that we blame mattresses for poor sleep quality when it's not always their fault. Poor mattresses. Now, if you're still sleeping on the hand-me-down twin mattress from your college dorm, then, Houston, we have a problem!

If you have the funds to spend on a mattress, and your mattress is over ten years old, then go shopping. Try out a lot of options. Innerspring, gel, memory foam, pillowtop, adjustable, and even waterbeds are just some of the mattresses available.

If you are able to go shopping, start the trip online. Look at the stores near you and read up on actual customer reviews of the mattresses available. Unfortunately, there is no consistency to the claims most mattress manufacturers make. They can say it is fluffy like a cloud and your spine will be perfectly aligned like your favorite constellation, but no one regulates those claims. Then, after you step into a mattress store, you have the very hard-working salespeople who can sway your decision.

Go in with a plan. Rest on each mattress for ten minutes. Type notes in your phone (or use a notebook if you prefer) about how you feel on each mattress. Then go home, research online some more, and plan to go back the next day. Giving your brain a night to think about a large purchase is always a good idea.

A good salesperson will try to create a feeling of scarcity. "This is the last one," or, "I had a couple looking at this mattress just this morning." Or maybe even, "This mattress is discontinued. Buy it now, or it will be gone forever!" I don't always remember to follow this wait-overnight advice, but it is the best plan. And I really want you to get your best sleep!

Sheets

Bedding needs to be clean and easily breathable. This is why cotton generally reigns supreme, although bamboo and silk are not bad options. Here are the questions that I had: If cotton is the best, why is some cotton so scratchy? Can I wash it over and over to make it softer?

Many experts agree that cotton is a great choice for sheets, but do you know how many types of cotton sheets there are? It is freaking overwhelming—Supima®, Pima, long staple, Egyptian—and this list is not even close to exhaustive because then you need to know about thread counts and weave.

Here's my advice because, like I said, I get overwhelmed. Go to a store, feel the sheets, buy what you like. I have found that buying Egyptian cotton gets me closer to a sheet that I like. Then, I must also remember not to buy the sateen weave that is too thick for my liking but great for cold sleepers and to look for deep pockets for my super thick Tempur-Pedic® memory foam mattress. I have had good luck and bad with sheets from Amazon, Overstock, and Macy's. That's why I recommend that you go to a store, feel them, and then purchase.

Pillows and the Best-Kept Secret of Pregnant Women

Pillows are the most important part of the entire process of setting up the ideal sleeping surface. Pillows come in as many sizes and shapes and flavors as you can imagine. I went with a shaped Tempur-Pedic® pillow, but you really need to try a few out to get your best fit.

Now for the best part. Go buy a body pillow if you don't have one! Supporting my entire body is a luxury that I now require. This could have something to do with the reconstructed chest that I have due to breast cancer, but whatever! I still think you should try out a body pillow. It may or may not work for you, but you won't know unless you try. I bought a cheap body pillow for only $10, and it works for me. If you want to see the variety available, type "best pregnancy body pillow" into any search engine and look around.

Tip

Sleeping surface options are unique to each individual. If you have a partner you are sharing your bed with, then you may want to look into the split mattress options that come with the adjustable beds. Then you could look at the Sleep Number beds that allow each side of the bed to be a totally different firmness. I am lucky because my husband and I each agreed on our current mattress, although we have had it for almost fifteen years. So we are in the market for a new one. Cross your fingers that we can agree on the next mattress. Or maybe we'll end up with the split mattress. Who knows?

Chapter 4—Temperature

Vasodilation: the widening of your blood vessels. It happens when smooth muscles found in the walls of arteries or large veins relax, allowing the blood vessels to become more open. This leads to an increase in blood flow through your blood vessels as well as a decrease in blood pressure.
—from Healthline

When you go to bed, are your hands and feet icicles? If you are reading this book, I am going to guess the answer is yes. Why?

Your body follows an internal biological process known as a circadian rhythm. This process follows the sun's rise and fall and is affected by light and temperature. We are warmer when we are awake and the sun is up and cooler when we are asleep and the sun has set.

Our bodies have a process that sends blood to the hands and feet to help cool our core temperature by a few degrees. This process is called vasodilation and should lead to warmer hands and feet as we fall asleep. If your hands and feet are cold, you may struggle to fall asleep. Maybe your body just sucks at vasodilation. I personally am convinced my body has a broken vasodilator. Ask my husband—warm hands and feet have *never* happened, much to his dismay.

Warm feet equals faster to sleep! And even though we want warm feet, we need the rest of our body to be at a cooler temperature for optimum sleep.

If you can afford another purchase, invest in a fan or AC unit specifically for your bedroom. Turn your bedroom thermostat a few degrees cooler. These steps may help your body get into a sleepy state. Most experts say 65–70 degrees is an optimal range for sleep, although your best temp may be a little higher or lower.

On the other hand, if you struggle to fall asleep, maybe you don't really know your optimal room temperature. Try a little action research and test strategies to figure out what works. Do not just keep doing what you have been doing if it's not working. We have all heard that definition of insanity—doing the same thing over and over and expecting different results.

Along with having cooler temperatures for sleep, watching what you do right before bed is important. Look at your pre-sleep activities in terms of body temperature. Super-hot baths or a HIIT workout will not help your body cool down. Leave at least an hour between heat-producing exercise or steamy showers and climbing under the covers. Also make sure your pajamas are conducive to lower body temperatures. That fleece onesie might not be the best choice.

Tip

Action research—in this case, a process to examine your own actions—is a great way to test a few options to help determine your best sleep temperature.

Be advised that your best sleep temperature also needs to take into account the pajamas, sheets, and blankets on your bed. The type of mattress that you have is also a factor. Many people dislike the memory foam mattresses because they form to your body. That offers great support, but it can also make you warmer, as the mattress is trapping some of your body heat.

Chapter 5—Journal

Trauma: the response to a deeply distressing or disturbing event that overwhelms an individual's ability to cope, causes feelings of helplessness, diminishes their sense of self and their ability to feel a full range of emotions and experiences.
—from Integrated Listening

Journaling is a required bedtime activity, but don't worry. I will share a journaling hack that will make it super quick. Read this list of possible benefits and select all that you think have been linked to journaling:

A. stress reduction
B. lower blood pressure
C. overall happiness
D. better sleep

If you guessed E: all of the above, you are the winner! Journaling makes you healthier. It's true! James W. Pennebaker, a researcher at the University of Texas at Austin, found that writing for fifteen to twenty minutes a day just three to five times over a four-month period was enough to lower blood pressure. So, based on that research, you may not even need to journal every day.

The rewards are the greatest if a specifically stressful or traumatic event happened. Other benefits include clearing your mind so you can wind down, allowing your thoughts to quiet.

Don't worry. This journaling doesn't require a complicated process, correct spelling, or perfect handwriting. The goal is to scoop the thoughts off the surface of your brain so you can shut it off for the night.

For some, this may only take two minutes. Others might spend at least five minutes. Just start writing and quit when your thoughts slow. It can be a recap of your day, but the benefits that we are seeking will increase if you choose to use this journaling time for two things.

First, write down three to five things you are grateful for. These can be as simple as a beautiful flower that you smelled or as complex as your marriage.

Second, write down your to-do list for tomorrow. Just jotting down the things you want to accomplish the next day allows your brain to let those things go. You have a plan, and it is written down, so you won't forget it. You can even take a picture of the list with your phone if you need to. It is amazing how just outlining the things you need to get done the next day will help you.

The main rule is to keep this journal right next to your bed. The journal needs to be one of the last things you do each night. If you journal too early, then your brain will come up with a whole new list to worry about, or at least that's what my brain does. The other reason that you need this next to your bed is for those pesky middle-of-the-night thoughts. Write them down so you can go back to sleep quickly!

Tip
If you had a terrible day or a really traumatic event happened, journal about that before dinner. This will give your body a chance to cool down after reliving all those feelings. Just save the three to five things you are grateful for and your to-do list for right before bed.

Note from Stephanie

You have now read the first part of *The Sleep Habit*, and you just finished reading about the importance of journaling. While you are in the writing mood and *before* you read the next really difficult part, would you consider going to Amazon and leaving a review? I am still very much a fledgling author, and reviews help so much! Thank you! And remember to go to StephanieEwingAuthor.com to pick up your #eat4sleep meal plan!

Part II
The Keys to Sleep

Your bedroom is ready. Now, we'll move on to the hardest and most important part of your new sleep habit. Stay committed.
Your sleep is important.
You are important.

Chapter 6—Touchy Subject

Cell phone addiction, sometimes referred to as problematic mobile phone use, is a behavioral addiction thought to be similar to that of an internet, gambling, shopping, or video game addiction and leads to severe impairment or distress in one's life.
—from PsychGuides

I am really sorry to have to address the cell phone glued to your hand, but it is necessary. Did you know that 60 percent of college students in the United States think they are addicted to their cell phones?

Let's convince ourselves that cell phones need to sleep too. Set up a family charging station in the kitchen.

Excuses (arguments that I have with myself):
- But I need to read to get sleepy.
  - Answer: Bust out your library card, or dust off an old favorite on the shelf. You should see my bookshelves! And I have a few that I've never read.

- But my phone is my alarm clock.
  - Answer: Buy an alarm clock.

- But I like to listen to a sleep story before bed.
  - Answer: Hmmm, maybe buy Bluetooth earbuds, turn on your sleep story from your phone in the kitchen, and listen in bed.

- But my work needs to be able to contact me.
  - Answer: When was the last time that happened? If this is true, you can create a cell phone cave in your bedroom, but your phone needs to be tucked into a tissue box so the phone will not be visible. Only get it out if work calls. You can set a special ringtone for work, and you'll always know if it's them.

- But I really like to play Yahtzee before bed.
  - Answer: Tough cookies. Do you want to sleep like a baby or play Yahtzee every night? I doubt the answer is Yahtzee if you purchased a book about sleep.

Cell phones are amazing tools and resources for us throughout our day. The ease of use and available information at our fingertips is truly awe-inspiring.

Cell phones are also very powerful devices that need to be treated with the care and concern of a ticking bomb. People of all ages are addicted to cell phones. People of all ages are addicted to online gambling and gaming. People of all ages are accessing pornography, and it is particularly damaging to developing young brains.

I had a colleague of mine in the school setting say, "Would you drop your child off at the local park at 10:00 pm?" The answer was a resounding no! Well, that is, in effect, what you are doing if you allow your child to be online unsupervised in their bedroom.

I get it. The whole process of writing a book, learning about marketing, using new social media outlets, creating book covers, collaborating with other authors, taking online courses—for me, this has increased my time on technology, and I wasn't at a low number to begin with. If you have an iPhone, go to **Settings** and scroll down to click **Screen Time**. At the time I am writing this book, my daily average screen time is two hours and four minutes.

Then click on the **More** arrow and look at how many times you pick up your phone to check it. This can be a crazy high number!

Even if you do not have any of the scary issues listed above, do you know the effects of screen time before bed? The National Sleep Foundation recommends that you stop using electronic devices, like your cell phone, at least thirty minutes before bedtime. Devices like your TV, cell phone, and laptop emit a bright blue light that mimics daylight in your brain. This messes up your melatonin levels and your circadian rhythm. Also, many times, the stuff we watch on those devices is very stimulating and may affect our adrenaline levels. This all leads to difficulty sleeping.

Not a tip, a requirement
Make your cell phone a bed, cave, house, or whatever you want to call it. Tell yourself that your cute little cell phone is a pet that needs to be cared for. This includes having its own space to rest. Put the damn thing to bed at least thirty minutes before you plan to go to bed.

This is the hardest step for me. I am thinking that I have a pretty serious case of too much cell phone use going on. For me, the way to fix this is by creating a habit that is easy to follow. First, I set a "downtime" in the **Screen Time** section under **Settings**. Then I created a charging station in the bathroom by my bedroom. This is still a struggle for me, and I am always finding new excuses for why my phone should be on my nightstand. Stay strong!

Chapter 7—Caffeine

Caffeine: a stimulant compound found naturally in coffee, tea, cocoa (chocolate), and kola nuts (cola) and added to soft drinks, foods, and medicines. Caffeine can cause anxiety, insomnia, nervousness, and hypertension. Caffeine is a diuretic and increases urination.
—from HealthNet

I am very skeptical of anyone who doesn't drink coffee. Just kidding. I am just jealous! However, caffeine intake needs to stop very early in the day in order to help your sleep.

Alcohol, diuretics, and spicy foods are also not great before bed. Many people—okay me. *I* included a glass of wine, a game on my phone, and maybe a book on my phone as a part of my ultimate bedtime routine. So, none of these things is recommended in this book. None of them work. The wine makes you pee and then feel dehydrated. The game on your phone and the book on your phone are both pretty stimulating, and the light on your phone is no good.

There's a reason so many people are making money selling blue-light blocking glasses. Yes, the blue light is affecting your circadian rhythm; however, the phone is a problem even without the blue light.

Having access to every bit of research, every dream destination, every fruit that starts with the letter p—having all these things at hand is not good. Yes, your brain will have random thoughts, but you do not need the ability to chase down every thought in the palm of your hand. That's why you now have a journal by your bed. If the thought is really nagging you, write it down. Look it up tomorrow.

Another problem with the cell phone is the ability to immediately purchase the next book in a series you're reading. This can drastically affect your sleep if it's a really great book series. I am an educator. I can always rationalize another book. They're good for our brains!

Tip

Enlist your partner or loved ones to help you stick to your new sleep habit. Create your "cell phone house" and put your cell phone to bed each night at the same time. Select your new "cell phone bedtime" in your downtime settings so your phone can tell you when to put it to bed!

Chapter 8—Consistency

Consistent: acting or done in the same way over time. —from Lexico

Here is another fact about sleep that I absolutely *hate*. I know that is a very strong word, but I believe there is a large percentage of you that will agree.

Here goes. In order to train ourselves to be able to fall asleep quickly, we need to be consistent. So far, so good. We will build a routine that allows us to get into the correct frame of mind to be sleepy. The part that I don't like is this: You need to do this at the same time each night, *and* you need to wake up at the same time each morning—seven days a week.

No sleeping in on the weekends. See? That sucks. But what I found that sucks even more is wasting years of my life trying to fall asleep instead of just falling asleep quickly and waking up feeling great.

This is just another part of my sleep habit that I struggle with, especially on Saturday mornings. The good news is that as I have gotten older, my need to pee in the morning helps ensure that I will wake up at a decent time. However, I still struggle not to climb right back into bed on Saturday mornings. I am definitely a work in progress. I just remind myself that going to sleep efficiently is an important skill that I am not very good at. I need to train myself to be better at this, and that includes waking up and staying up on

Saturday mornings. I use one of my techniques from *The Shower Habit* and set a reward for myself. Hmmm, dark chocolate. You can pick your own reward!

Tip

I had to do some more research on this consistency idea before I included it in this book. Unfortunately, our circadian rhythm once again plays a huge role in our ability to sleep. You may want to consider buying a light therapy box or sunrise alarm clock. Setting the same wake-up time each day has a *huge* impact. According to verywellhealth.com, the benefits include:

- Waking up easier
- Diminishing morning sleep inertia
- Falling asleep easier (less insomnia)
- Decreasing sleep deprivation
- Needing fewer naps
- Reducing caffeine dependence
- Improving alertness
- Sharpening focus and short-term memory
- Having a brighter mood
- Being less irritable
- Minimizing pain
- Boosting immune system function
- Performing safely on the job
- Driving safely and attentively

After reading all the benefits of waking up at the same time, I was sold. It had to become one of the foundations of a better sleep habit. Try it if you want to have improved sleep. C'mon, it's good for you!

Part III

Okay, the toughest part of your sleep habit is behind you. The rest is all downhill. You've got this!

Chapter 9—Herbal Tea and Pajamas

Decision fatigue occurs when people feel exhausted from making too many choices. By limiting how many inconsequential decisions we need to make and scheduling decision-making for times when we feel most alert, we may be able to make better decisions.
—from ThoughtCo

To successfully change your behavior, you need to make the new behavior the path of least resistance. If changing into your pajamas signals the start of your new bedtime routine, then make sure you lay your pjs on your bed after you make it in the morning.

If a nice warm cup of herbal tea is the next step after putting on your pajamas, then purchase the tea and have it in the cupboard next to the mugs. Even better, put a mug and a bag of tea on the counter when you get home from work.

This way, you have a visual reminder in your kitchen to drink your tea and another visual reminder in your bedroom with your pjs on your bed. This keeps it fresh in your mind and takes away the need to make a decision. By the end of the day, heck by mid-morning, sometimes you have already made so many tough decisions that your brain just gets tired and says, "Screw it!" Then you do whatever sounds good in the moment rather than thinking about your plans or long-term goals.

If you are stressed, tired, and facing decision fatigue, I can guarantee that, without some pretty clear, easy choices already lined up and set right in front of your face, you are going to choose instant gratification. That bag of chips from the vending machine or the 32 oz Pepsi from the gas station is going to end up happening.

Then you will feel bad about the choices, and the downward cycle continues. Your subconscious perks up and starts in on the negative self-talk and limiting beliefs, and a poor self-image becomes the focus. You can stop this cycle by making plans and creating habits.

Choosing a nighttime drink that helps you sleep is our next task. Have you tried all of these choices?

- Warm milk
- Almond milk
- Valerian tea
- Chamomile tea
- Tart cherry juice
- Passion fruit tea
- Peppermint tea

This list is nighttime approved to have within an hour of your bedtime. If you are not sure which drink you will enjoy, experiment. Does a warm drink or cold drink sound better? After making that decision, purchase a few choices and try each one before bed for the next week. The exact beverage doesn't matter. The routine of having an approved drink before bed does.

This is one more signal to your brain that will happen every time before bed. As this becomes ingrained in your evening ritual, your brain and body will begin reacting more and more favorably to the steps in your process of winding down from the day. It's like when the smell of sunscreen and the act of putting on a swimsuit, life vest, and sunglasses evokes excitement in a person who loves boating.

Now for some of the science behind why these drinks are approved for your nighttime routine. Chamomile tea has often been a first choice to those who want to sleep. It is thought that the antioxidant apigenin found in chamomile works with receptors in your brain that reduce anxiety. Valerian root has antioxidants that inhibit the amygdala, which processes strong emotion, thereby inducing calmness. The rest of the bunch either have melatonin in them or work with your body to produce melatonin.

Your body naturally produces melatonin, and it is at its highest levels about two hours before your sleep cycle. To help your body produce melatonin, make sure to get some natural sunlight during the day.

Tip

Buy a special sleepy time mug, especially for your sleepy time drink. My favorite mugs are made by Rae Dunn, and many have sayings on them. You can combine your sleep habit with an affirmation on your mug. Mine says, "You Got This." After you find your drink of choice, stock up and be consistent. Remember, we are creating a routine of actions in order to adopt a healthy sleep habit.

Chapter 10—Stretch

Flexibility: the quality of bending easily without breaking. —from Oxford Languages

Here's a fun challenge! Set your timer for every three hours. Each time you hear the chimes, stand up and stretch. Remember to lower your tongue from the roof of your mouth, unclench your jaw, drop your shoulders, and turn your head from side to side. Getting your blood pumping to loosen up tense muscles is beneficial and feels great all day long. Stretching before bed is an excellent choice to add to your very own bedtime routine.

Remember, we are working on creating your own personalized sleep habit that will help you to be an improved sleeper. Sleeping is a skill, and we are growing our sleeping toolbox. This book is your sleep tune-up. Ha! I'm really getting into this metaphor.

Back to why stretching should be a part of your evening. Focusing on your body and breath takes your mind off the details of your day. This change in focus helps your mind, and the stretching will reduce the likelihood of nighttime muscle cramps.

Speaking of cramps, my maternity class instructor recommended mustard as a muscle cramp reliever. It works! If you are experiencing a nighttime muscle cramp, hobble to the kitchen and squirt a bunch of mustard in your mouth. Boom! The cramp will be gone. Then drink a glass of water and go back to bed.

These are four great stretches to include in your winding-down routine:

1. Calf stretches—put your left toe on the wall and keep your heel on the floor. Stretch and hold for fifteen seconds. Repeat with your right foot.

2. Bear hug—stand tall and inhale as you open your arms wide, exhale, and cross your arms right over left and hug yourself. Hold for fifteen seconds. Inhale again as you open your arms wide, and exhale as you cross your arms left over right, hug yourself, and hold for fifteen seconds.

3. Seated forward bend—sit on the floor or your bed (not near the edge) with your legs stretched out in front of you and tuck your chin to your chest. Bend forward and reach for your toes. Hold for fifteen seconds.

4. Neck stretches—sit down and bring your left ear to your left shoulder and count five deep breaths. Do the same on the right side. Next, look to your left and hold for five breaths and then look right and hold for five breaths.

Tip

Many gentle stretches can feel good and help you decompress before bed. The only rule is that you should not be sweating, and you should focus on deep breaths and slow, gentle stretches that feel good, or hurt good, so to speak.

Chapter 11—Mindfulness

Mindfulness: a mental state achieved by focusing one's awareness on the present moment while calmly acknowledging and accepting one's feelings, thoughts, and bodily sensations; used as a therapeutic technique.
—from Oxford Languages

Practicing mindfulness before bed is another must-have step to your sleep habit. I am going to walk you through a basic mindfulness exercise that will allow your brain to focus on the present, letting go of the day and staying focused on where you are in this exact moment.

This technique can be used in a variety of settings and is very helpful for your brain. For any of you who used glitchy computers a decade ago like me, this is the control-alt-delete reset for your brain. It closes all your open browser tabs and cleans the slate, hopefully allowing your brain to run smoothly and focus on the current task, which is to become sleepy.

Do you find it ironic that we tell ourselves to wake up, quit yawning, and stay alert all day, and then when we are finally free to nod off, we freeze and can't do it? So annoying!

Okay, in a perfect world, you are reading this (paperback version) right before bed. So, dim your lamp, nestle into your mattress, and take a deep breath. Release the tension in your jaw and neck and lower your shoulders. Let your facial muscles relax and focus on your breath. Begin by counting to four as you inhale through your nose. Pause and count to five as you exhale out your mouth. Repeat that three times.

Now, be still and let your thoughts float through your mind like clouds in the sky. Tense and release your muscles, starting with your head and jaw. Tense those muscles, hold for ten seconds, and release those muscles as you exhale slowly. Tense and release the muscles of your neck and shoulders, your back and stomach, and finally your glutes and legs. Keep your breathing slow and deep.

You can also sit in silence and just focus on your breathing. There are so many helpful ways to practice mindfulness. Hopefully, you have already tried a few. This habit of focusing your mind on your breath and letting your thoughts float on by is a great stress reliever. The benefits of mindfulness are well documented.

Tip

I told you about this in *The Shower Habit*, and here it is again. I super love the Calm app. My favorite sleep meditation is called Deep Sleep Release, and it is twenty-five minutes long.

Chapter 12—Apps

Sleep stories: a Google search turns up almost two billion results in under a second. Go search and find a sleep story to listen to each night. Or you can search for a sleep meditation and choose one of those.

Have you ever listened to a sleep story? It's like having a bedtime story read to you as an adult. It is awesome! There are so many choices too. Do you want a deep voice or melodic voice to read to you? Do you like trains? Choose one of those.

Your homework is to check out a few sleep stories on an app like Calm or on YouTube. Just type "sleep stories" into a search engine and listen to a few. When you find one you like, bookmark it, text yourself the link, or write it down. Tonight, try out the story. Remember those Bluetooth earbuds because your phone will not be in the same room as you. Or yell, "Alexa, play a sleep story!" Caution: If you don't actually own an Amazon device, your family *will* look at you funny.

I look for soothing voices and repetitive words with stories about sleep and finding sleep. Definitely choose a voice that sounds relaxing to you. I also choose one that is thirty minutes or less.

Tip
Think of your favorite actor or singer and go search
for their name plus "sleep story." Many famous people
have recorded sleep stories, and you can find them
on YouTube.

Chapter 13—Partners

I want to give you actionable tips for dealing with someone else in the bed. I also want to share with you a new trend of separate beds or separate blankets or even a "sleep divorce."

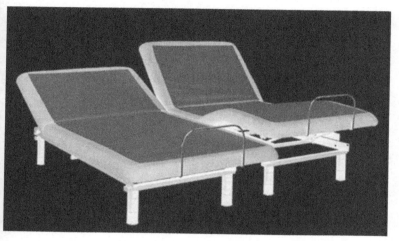

The Scandinavian sleep method involves one mattress, two blankets, two happy sleepers. Each couple has just one bed, but there are two comforters. That way, no one person can be a blanket hog, and you can have different levels of warmth for each sleeper.

Having separate beds is another new trend that is actually an old trend. Historically, only poor people slept in the same bed because they couldn't afford more space. Rich people each had their own beds and bedrooms. The current trend can involve the same bedroom with two separate beds like a double queen hotel room. Or this can involve a full "sleep divorce" when each person gets a separate bed in a separate bedroom. Depending on whether your partner snores, needs a radio on, or has some other sleep-disturbing activity, you may want to consider your sleeping options.

Tip
The Ikea furniture store has a lot of sleep options. If you live close to an Ikea, you can go wander through the store and check out all the fully furnished bedroom areas.

Chapter 14—Flying First Class

What do the airlines get right? Masks? Earplugs? Washcloths? Socks? At least the airlines do this in first class.

Okay, truth-time. I have not flown first-class. But I did once get to fly business-first, and that was really freaking awesome! Here is what I found out: Airplanes know how to promote sleep better than many of us right now.

As I entered the plane bound for Amsterdam from Chicago, I was handed a little zippered pouch with the airline's logo as I sat down in my large recliner-style seat with the fold-up TV in the armrest. It was pretty darn comfortable, and it almost fully reclined. Now, my hubby was used to flying like this for his work. I was not. The entire experience was almost surreal.

After I opened the little pouch, I pulled out a sleep mask, earplugs, earbuds, socks, and hand lotion. Wow! Everything that would help me sleep on this overnight flight to Europe. With my feet warm, my eyes totally covered, and my earplugs in place, I slept very well. I am sure the previous week of wedding-related activities followed by the actual wedding, reception, and well-wishes from all our loved ones also added to my ability to sleep. However, you can't discount warm feet, pleasantly scented lotion, no light or sound, and a comfy recliner!

When was the last time you spent money on your own sleep? You need to sleep in order to stay alive. You will spend over thirty *years* of your life asleep. Now, the time you spend falling asleep is time that can be better spent either sleeping or living. Trying to fall asleep is wasted time. That can add up to seven or more *years* of an average life. Let's work on that.

Tip
During my research for this book, I went to a couple of airlines to check out what I was missing in First Class nowadays. My one-time experience was over twenty years ago. Turns out, the names have all changed, and now First Class sounds like Deluxe Comfort Extraordinaire Plus-Plus. Also, the little pouch that I remember is now called an amenity kit. And for Delta Airlines, it's in a Tumi zippered bag! As Fancy Nancy would say, "Ooh-la-la!"

Chapter 15—Daily Sleep-Adjacent Activities

Neuroscience of sleep is the study of the neuroscientific and physiological basis of the nature of sleep and its functions. The importance of sleep is demonstrated by the fact that organisms daily spend hours of their time in sleep, and that sleep deprivation can have disastrous effects, ultimately leading to death. —Wikipedia entry for the Neuroscience of Sleep

It's no question that exercise is good for you, but did you realize the important part that some form of daily exercise plays in your sleep? Exercise during the day leads to better sleep. In order to make this chapter accessible to the most people, we are going to focus on increasing our step count.

So, what's the deal with 10,000 steps every day? Why is the 10,000-step goal so specific? Is it really that important? Yes and no.

First, let's talk about the benefits of 10,000 steps daily. It's a nice round number that's easy to remember, and many of our step-counting devices automatically come preset to that number. More steps every day may lead to a longer life span. Walking helps build muscle, improve heart and lung function, and stabilize blood sugar because your muscles use more of the glucose in your blood.

You may be shocked to learn that the specific 10,000-step mark is a little arbitrary. In fact, simply *increasing* the number of steps you take every day is an excellent goal. Getting to a baseline of 7,500 steps every day has proven health benefits. Walking or getting exercise daily improves your mood and boosts your energy.

A little digging around shows the possible origins of the magic number 10,000. It turns out that in 1965, a Japanese company sold a pedometer called Manpo-kei, which translates directly to "10,000 steps meter." This all happened around the Olympic Games, and we all know we go a little crazy around that time. Hello, *Cool Runnings* Jamaican luge team? So, 10,000 steps is a little bit arbitrary, but getting 7,500 steps or more steps than you currently get— those are significant targets to aim for.

The American Heart Association recommends the following:

- Get at least 150 minutes per week of moderate-intensity aerobic activity or 75 minutes per week of vigorous aerobic activity, or a combination of both, preferably spread throughout the week.
- Add moderate- to high-intensity muscle-strengthening activity, such as resistance or weights, at least two days per week.

- Spend less time sitting. Even light-intensity activity can offset some of the risks of being sedentary.
- Gain even more benefits by being active at least 300 minutes (5 hours) per week.
- Increase amount and intensity gradually over time.

Knowing your current level of physical activity and gradually increasing it will lead to a longer life and better sleep!

Tip

Tracking your minutes of exercise or your steps will help keep your exercise goal at the front of your mind. Standing more than you are sitting, wearing your tennis shoes, and wearing a step-counting device can all help you on the road to better sleep and better health in general.

I read in my chiropractor's office, "Sitting for your spine is like sugar for your teeth." After you eat sugar, brush your teeth. After you sit for a prolonged period, stretch and go for a walk. We've got this.

Chapter 16—Settling on Your Sleep Routine

Habit stacking is the idea that by clustering the habits we want to develop and sustain, we stand more chance of remembering them by associating related tasks with each other.
—from journalist Steve Scott

We have covered most of the most beneficial things you can do to improve your sleep. One last recommendation involves a bath or shower. Many experts encourage you to take a bath or shower to help you relax before bed. If a bath or shower is a part of your bedtime routine, make sure it's not too hot. A warm or warm-hot shower or bath is relaxing and helpful. If it's too hot, it increases your body temperature, and that is not what you need for bedtime. Your body works to cool you off for optimum sleep.

The only way these steps will work is if you do them consistently. We need to engage our brain's love of routines and ability to predict next steps. If we consistently engage in specific habits before bed, our brains will predict that we are getting ready to sleep. Then it will increase melatonin production, start the vasodilation process, and make us feel snoozy!

Sample Bedtime Routine:
- Eat4Sleep dinner
- Body pillow
- Nightstand with journal
- Cell phone on charger in kitchen one hour before bed
- Warn cup of tea
- Stretch
- Sleep story
- Turn down thermostat
- Journal: gratitude and to-do list for tomorrow
- Meditate: breathing exercise
- Get in comfy bed
- Fall asleep

Chapter 17—Final Challenge: Gain 3 Years of Life

Gamification: taking something that is not a game and applying game mechanics to increase user engagement, happiness, and loyalty. —from Growth Engineering

Have you heard the term gamification? Okay, here's an easier one. Have you heard of Candy Crush? Candy Crush is the definition of how a game can use psychology to keep us motivated to continue playing, spend money, and feel great about it. An everyday example for me is the coffee shop stamp card. That's a good one!

Here is the reason I chose my very first topic to write a book about to be waking up happy. The second book, which you are now reading, is all about finding a consistent routine to allow you to sleep soundly. I believe that great sleep and a motivating morning routine are together the foundation for you to accomplish *all* your dreams.

Thank you for coming along with me on this journey. If you are implementing the habits you are reading about, you are beginning to see a drastic increase in your energy and vastly improved mindset. And I believe you are poised to take off. What area of life are you going to focus on next? Your career, your health, your relationships—anything your heart desires—because if you change something you do every day, you are incrementally building an entirely new future.

Take charge of your life and consciously direct your subconscious. Let your imagination go and tap into your reticular activating system. This system is running at all times and will be working for you whether you are actively thinking about your goals or not. You just need to do the work to become clear on what your goals are. This tells your system what to be on the lookout for!

Have you ever started researching a new car that you want to buy? Let's say that you decide you want to purchase a vintage Volkswagen Beetle. Something crazy will happen. You will begin seeing VW bugs everywhere! Now, were all these gems hiding in garages and are just now out driving around tempting you because you want to buy one? Or have all these cool cars been there the entire time, and your brain was just filtering them out of your consciousness because they didn't mean anything to you?

I am thinking this is not a case of magic VW Beetles coming to life just to taunt you. You decided on a goal. You researched that goal. And now your subconscious is giving you what you want more of. Use this magic for your own good.

Get clear on your dreams. Research them. Buy books about them and join Facebook groups dedicated to your dreams. Talk to people who have done what you are dreaming about doing. Just like Winnie the Pooh says, "You are braver than you believe, stronger than you seem, and smarter than you think."

Action to take in the next 5 minutes:

You need to daydream. What huge hairy goals have been percolating in the back on your mind? Marathons, mountain climbing, traveling, writing, painting, starting a business, joining a dating site, photography—do any of these thoughts make you smile, give you butterflies, or evoke any other strong emotions?

Start with those. Sketch, journal, dance, dream, research, and then decide on the dream you are going to pursue. This is only the first dream you are going to tackle. After reading this book and creating the sleep habit that works the best for you, you will be gaining back up to seven years of your life that you would have spent trying to fall asleep. What are you going to do with seven years? Not seven days, not seven weeks, we are talking over three million minutes! How about holding a plank for a minute? With an additional three million minutes, do you think you could change the shape of your physical fitness? How about writing for a minute? Could you write a book? The possibilities are only limited by your imagination and the actions you take every day. Are your wheels turning? Are you inspired? Awesome! Now go back and reread this book and begin taking action.

For the skeptics:

Okay, if you are a mathematician and a skeptic, let's complete a story problem together. Let's say, like me, you are 45 years old. Half of your life is already behind you. So you can't really gain back all seven years that the average person spends falling asleep. Now, we are working with three and a half years. Let's round down and say three years. Now, instant sleep is not a reality unless you are my husband, so let's say you only improve your falling asleep time by 50 percent. Now, we're talking about one and a half years. Okay, you got me, you now only have 788,000 extra minutes. I bet writing or planking or running for 788,000 minutes wouldn't do anything to change your life. Well, I guess you may as well not even try....

Sarcasm, I know. If your glass is half full, you believe that you now have an additional 3 million minutes. If your glass is half empty, you only have half a million minutes. That is just the extra time you would have already spent falling asleep. We haven't even touched the 300,000 minutes you already get to spend every year of your life. Are there other issues with my math story problem? Probably. I'm sorry, Mrs. Gary, I have not kept up with my algebra homework every day.

Bottom line: You have the time. You have the energy. Go do something that sounds really hard!

For the Soon-To-Be Weird People:

If you follow the sleep habit steps, you might find that your creativity spikes right before you fall asleep. This is a great thing, but you are going to need to have that journal right next to your bed so you can track those amazing ideas. Those ideas have been percolating in your mind the entire time, but you were not aware of them until you created the space to pay attention. Once you create the space in your life for your mind to do what it does best, which is create, then you are going to see this hour before bedtime as an amazing part of your day.

One of my idols, Dave Ramsey, says that being weird means you have to do things differently than normal people. Spoiler alert: both Dave and I recommend you try to be weird because normal is really out-of-whack. In order for this to make sense, we need to define the difference between weird and normal as it relates to the sleep habit we are trying to create.

Normal = Tired

If you don't mind being tired, never having enough time to accomplish your goals, and being really good at games on your phone, then go ahead. Be normal! Continue wasting time on your phone and watch your screen time continue to rise as the years roll by. To achieve expert levels of normalness, play a bunch of games on your phone and scroll through social media right before bed. Then immediately before you lie down, drink caffeine or alcohol. These things will almost ensure a less-than-stellar night's sleep. And guess what, most "normal people" are not getting the quality or quantity of sleep they need so they can be at their best physically, mentally, or emotionally.

Be weird.

Weird people can be almost militant in their zest to accomplish the routines that allow them to be the healthiest. Tracking their steps, installing apps on their phones to create tech-free time before bed, not eating or snacking two to three hours before bed … Geez, those weirdos! Well, here is the deal. If you are a Dave Ramsey weirdo, you have *zero* debt. If you are a Sleep Habit weirdo, you feel rested. Are you beginning to see the benefits of weirdness?

Keep reading for a day-by-day summary of your new sleep habit!

Day 1 of Your Sleep Habit

Consider planning a sleepy time meal high in melatonin.

Must do

Go to your sleeping space and clear off and clean your nightstand. Put a journal, pen, lip balm, nail clippers, glass of water (basically all the things that could require you to get out of bed) on your nightstand.

Consider your sleeping surfaces. Wash your sheets, buy a new pillow if you don't like the one you have, and really consider buying a body pillow.

Consider your optimum sleeping temperature, adjust as you are able to create the best sleep environment.

Must do

Right before bed, write down three things you are grateful for and create a list of your to-dos for the next day.

Must do

put your cell phone on its charger (not in your bedroom) at least thirty minutes before sleep.

Must do

End all caffeine intake before lunch. Consider waking up at the same time every single day.

Consider setting out your pajamas and herbal tea or bedtime-approved drink in the morning so you will be prepared for your nighttime routine.

Consider stretching, meditating, listening to a sleep story or other calming activity.

Consider setting an exercise or step goal to help your new sleep habit.

Must do

Write your new sleep habit steps in the front of your journal. Keep revising your list as needed.

Day 2 of Your Sleep Habit

Must Do

Go to your sleeping space, clear off and clean the nightstand. Put a journal, pen, lip balm, nail clippers, glass of water (basically all the things that could require you to get out of bed) on your nightstand.

Right before bed, write down three things you are grateful for and create a list of your to-dos for the next day.

Put your cell phone on its charger (not in your bedroom) at least thirty minutes before sleep.

End all caffeine intake before lunch.

Write your new sleep habit steps in the front of your journal. Keep revising as needed.

Consider planning a trip to a mattress, bedding, or pillow store. Your new body pillow is calling you.

Consider stopping by the grocery store and picking up some of your favorite foods from the sleepy foods list.

Read back through the book. Did you need to pick up a new alarm clock, phone charging station or a Rae Dunn mug with an affirmation?

Day 3 of Your Sleep Habit:

Think through your struggle points from the first two days. What do we need to tweak in order to make your new sleep habit really successful? You could be considering some pretty major changes to your lifestyle at this point. Do you need to cut back on the evening drinks? Do you need to really watch your cell phone usage? Are you considering spending big bucks on a new bed? Maybe your physical health and steps per day are your focus. Whatever your need, make a plan, lay out the things needed as a visual reminder, and choose a lead measure that you are going to track. If it is steps per day, then create a bait tracker chart with three checkboxes per day:

- ☐ I packed my tennis shoes and socks in a bag to take to work.
- ☐ I went for a walk at lunch.
- ☐ I made my step goal for the day.

See how many days in a row you can meet these three goals!

A happier, healthier you is just three days away. We can do this together. My Sleep Habit is a continual work in progress, improving every day! Keep tracking your lead measures and celebrating your small wins. You Got This!

Note from the Author

I greatly appreciate your time reading or listening to this book. I hope you have created your own personalized sleep habit and are on track to a well-rested and healthier you! If you have not already, go read *The Shower Habit* for help creating an amazing morning routine.

Remember to visit StephanieEwingAuthor.com for free resources.

I also would absolutely love it if you would take a few minutes to leave a review on Amazon. I want to help as many people as possible achieve healthy sleep habits. Reviews help this book reach more readers. I would also really like to hear your questions or comments. Your honesty will help me write even better books for you. I also would love to hear about what area of your life I should research next. Let's collaborate!

Thank you,

Stephanie

Made in the USA
Monee, IL
10 October 2023

44361521R00046